THE PHYSICS OF QI

Soko Paul Karsten

For:

Heze

With Deep Gratitude to:

Joshu, Leonard, & Molly

CONTENTS

Title Page   1

Dedication   3

                                            5

Prologue   7

Chapter 1 - Realization   13

Chapter 2 - Education   27

Qi Exercise #1   39

Chapter 3 - Transformation   44

Chapter 4 - Zero   52

Qi Exercise #2   63

Chapter 5 - Come Healing   72

Qi Exercise #3   85

Final Thoughts   95

                                           97

Appendix   97

References   101

Contact   103

About The Author   105

                                          107

PROLOGUE

What is Qi?

Imagine that there is a fundamental principle in our cosmos. One that is present with the very tiniest of moments and particles, and one that is apparent in the largest expanses of galaxies throughout our universe. Imagine this is an activity that expands and contracts, appears and disappears, turns negative and positive, and in essence is the rhythmic basis for the construct of everything we experience; be it the sun shining, a mosquito flying, or your thoughts on the matter.

The Chinese observed this dynamic throughout their lives, the expansion/contraction and wave like phenomena of the activities of nature, the cyclical coming and going of processes on the earth as well as in the heavens. They also experienced it within their bodies with the sensation of the breath, the heart beat, the regularity of the digestive system, the periods of sleep and awakening, the movements and flows of their bodies and emotions. With living and dying. This activity they named Qi.

No one knows why, but the common denominator of our universe is that everything, material and energetic, oscillates in this contracting/expanding way at the primal level, forming waves and vibrations that generate existence as we know it. So Qi itself is not physical, or non-physical. Yet it is the basis of everything physical and non-physical. It is the infinitely expanding/contracting principle that simply is. Everything manifests this Qi activity.

Quantum physics recognizes this phenomena in its discovery that the expanses of our universe, and hence our existence, are in essence a sea, a primordial soup of vibrating energetic phenomena that expand/contract, appear/disappear, and sometimes transcend time and space, making the primal aspect of our whole cosmos a chaotic ocean of possibilities. This science states that at the root our atoms, our cells, our tissues, organs, bodies, and minds are frequency-based facets of beingness intertwined with and interconnected with our vibratory environment and the universe at large. That life is a symphony of expanding/contracting activities that generate form and energy in a way that looks solid and somewhat fixed to us, but at its source is anything but.

This can be difficult for our minds to accept and grasp, particularly if our only view and experience of reality is that we are all inherently autonomous people with individual minds, separate from physical objects and our environment. But some of the ancients, and not so ancient Chinese, and others around the globe in various eras, found that if we open up to experiencing the fundamental principle in our universe, what the Chinese call Qi, we are provided with a glimpse and feel of this interconnected realm science states exists at our core and all around us.

When we do this, it is also found we subjectively experience feeling more peaceful and connected to others, and have more understanding of ourselves and our universe as a whole. But we also discover that the more disconnected we feel from this experience of Qi flow and vibration; the more we then experience personal suffering and illness, as well as a sense of separation and cognitive rigidity regarding those around us.

Therefore East Asian health practices over the centuries focused on becoming more aware of and developing physical exercises and modalities that support this universally shared Qi activity. This reconnecting our awareness and life practices with these natural rhythms enhance a sense of personal well being, and a deeper understanding of our "original" self. That is a connectivity with the natural world and cosmos that surrounds us.

In summary, the expansive/contractive activity we all share, regardless of if we are energy or matter, formless or formed, conscious or unconscious, living or inanimate, we call Qi.

CHAPTER 1 - REALIZATION

It was 1996 when a young scientist specializing in neuroanatomy and working in a laboratory on human brain research and dysfunction woke up with a severe headache. Over the next several hours she watched as her "normal" self of being a well-educated and busy individual gradually disappeared and was replaced by a pervasive pixillated universe of infinite energy in which there existed no time and space or person, but instead a sense of presence, of a flowing and connecting together into a realm of experience she later would term "la la land".

That morning her cognitive self, that was slipping away, did recognize that she was having a brain dysfunction of her own, a stroke.

And that the bleeding was located in the left side of her brain and was therefore shutting down her mental capacities for linear rational thought, personal history, and sense of time. Fortunately she was able to recognize the symptoms in time to have sufficient clarity to call colleagues for help and get transported to the hospital.

The experience of losing connection with her individual identity while opening up to an experience of immense connectivity with the universe had a transformative effect on her. So after a significant recovery time Jill Bolte Taylor wrote a book on her experience called *My Stroke of Insight*, and appeared on a Ted Talk with the same title. You can view this 19 minute video on You Tube at this link:

https://www.ted.com/talks/
jill_bolte_taylor_my_stroke_of_insight

Jill describes the differences of her experiences; the one being that of an individualized autonomous thinking being, and the other being that of a cosmic flow of the universe fundamentally filled with goodwill. She explains that they represent two very different functions of the left and right hemispheres of the brain. These two hemispheres have very different kinds of neural and physiological connections and programming, and therefore experience the world and life in very different ways. She stated in her talk that she believes that we can consciously choose which side of the brain we are going to act from. She also believes it is important to develop the right side of our brain, the side that provides access to the expansive/contractive interconnected energy of the universe, the side of our selves that experiences the reality of the connection we share together.

Jill's realization regarding her brain hemispheres points at a fundamental aspect of nature and reality as we now know it. Quantum physics, particularly due to the observations and insights of one of its most famous scientists, Neils Bohr, postulates that the very basis of our reality is formed through binaries. That is two, often opposing and independent looking qualities, that are actually polar aspects of a whole that interact in order to make up the whole, and therefore form reality.

Neils named this binary activity complementarity, and stated it was a core element to all of quantum reality, and therefore our existence. Further, scientists discovered that the more you tried to understand and measure one of these polar aspects of quantum binaries, the more invisible the other aspect became, and thus the more uncertain the outcome of your findings. In fact, that it was impossible to know the whole, or either of the binaries with certainty.

This led to the understanding that in the quantum world, there are not certainties, there are at best probabilities. That underlying our sense of physical order in the world we believed exists, is a chaotic universe that does not abide by the Newtonian laws of nature. This is the basis for Heisenberg's formulation of the Uncertainty Principle. To get the best sense of clarity within this fuzzy universe, scientists found they had to sit somewhere in the middle, between the two polar aspects of the binaries and, sort of, out of the corners of their eyes, observe both aspects simultaneously.

But even this did not provide the kind of certainty that scientists had gotten used to within the world of Newtonian physics and the physical realm that we normally think of with fixed time and space and the laws of nature.

Jill directly experienced this dualistic reality. On the one side she experienced herself as a particulate individual, having seemingly fixed attributes in time and space in this world, as well as being an accomplished neuroanatomist. On the other hand, she experienced her self as having no body, no history, no separation from the flow of energy in the universe, and felt a euphoric sense of liberation with this interconnectivity.

But it was not only quantum physics or Jill's personal experience with the left and right brain differences that have described this binary activity in our existence. The definition of a dialectic is a perspective that holds two seemingly contradictory or opposite ideas, that are, instead of being separate, believed to be two polar aspects of a whole. And thus problem solving or the study of reality using this approach hold that these oppositional forces are not independent and separate entitites. This method looks at the middle dynamic that holds the contradiction of the plurality of possibilities, while also finding the places where they meet or are useful. This is akin to the understanding of reality in ancient China, that perceived the world as being made up of inter-dependent opposites that transformed into each other in order to form reality. This Chinese version is called Yin/Yang theory.

So coming full circle, we find that the ancient Chinese, like quantum physicists, observed an expansive/contractive activity that formed reality and used a binary approach to understand the whole. The Chinese named their binary approach yin/yang theory and the fundamental expansive/contractive activity of reality as Qi.

Briefly, some attributes observed in the natural world and associated with yang are expansion, heat, light, positive, movement and life. And the observed phenomena associated with yin include contraction, cold, dark, negative, substance and death. These are commonly held versions of yin/yang attributes. *Note that I did not attribute good or bad to one or the other of these aspects.* The two are considered equal, and both necessary for existence, as in exhalation and inhalation. Chinese thought looked at how these qualities were interdependent, transforming back and forth into each other, and as such describing the activity of Qi, that is the cycles, rhythms and oscillatory phenomena of nature.

This way of knowing was also applied to understanding human health and is the basis for acupuncture, qi gong, and other modalities in East Asian Medicine. In this applied version of understanding the Qi activity, health practitioners seek to discover the balance and harmony of the yin/yang dynamic in the body to promote a sense of well being. Thus the history of yin/yang theory is a study of the interdependence and harmony of the two seemingly oppositional functions that make up Qi.

Now switching back to quantum physics; what further research has shown is that these binaries often register on one hand as being particulate, seemingly intentional fixed "objects" or entities, and on the other hand as having no fixed state, but appearing more as an expansive/contractive chaotic wave, quantum field, or the cosmos itself. As we heard above, this was the experience of Jill Bolte Taylor when she suffered her stroke. So we are seeing that this dualistic nature of the activity is not isolated to quantum reality, but also shows up in our "Newtonian" physical world as well.

Therefore the two disciplines from East and West find common ground in that this expansive/contractive activity is found, behind the curtain so to speak, embedded in all aspects of our existence, being the fundamental quality of the makeup of our cosmos.

This became acutely demonstrated to quantum physicists with the results of the famous, or infamous, double slit experiment.

It was in this experiment that the dualistic reality of photons (light) was demonstrated. The research showed that on one hand a photon acts as a particle, a discrete packet of specific frequency; but on the other hand it acts just as happily as a wave, or even a whole ocean, invisible to researchers, but demonstrated by the math and the final outcomes. (See the backplate of this little book. Also note in references at the end of this text a little animated video on this experiment that is on You Tube).

At the time that these experimental results were reported, many physicists were in disbelief because they had been brought up learning that in reality something was either eternally a particle, or a wave, but not both. What was even more disconcerting was that in an additional stage of the double slit experiment the very act of trying to measure or see how or when the photon transformed from particle to wave or wave to particle caused the photon to stop its transformative activity! So the photon even seemed to sense the desire to understand it, and in its shyness, refused to accommodate the research, and collapsed into its particulate state. And this was hard core science.... Take a moment to view the video listed in the reference section and contemplate the results of this experiment and how it matches, or doesn't match, your belief and experience of reality.

So what is appearing is that these binaries, in addition to appearing contradictory, or opposites, are also exhibiting the properties of being particulate in one state, and infinitely wave-like and infinitely expanding/contracting in the other state - yet both states are required to make up the whole. Thus all of you, since you are from the ground up composed of these incredibly small photons and electrons and quarks and such, manifest both individualized and formless selves. It is not just the right and left hemispheres of your brain that exhibit this dichotomy - it is every one of the trillions and trillions of atomic particles and energy packets and vibrations that make up your existence that exhibit this binary "droplet / ocean" function. Also note your intention to become self aware and observe this would/could shut down the whole transformative process of the particle/wave function (at least temporarily) according to the findings of the Double Slit Experiment. You are both the droplet tossed out of the ocean momentarily, and the ocean itself that you, the droplet, return to.

Though this may cognitively appear counter-intuitive or at least mysterious to the rational mind, it is a fundamental understanding of the nature of this activity if studied from the perspective of experiencing Qi. I remember reading a book entitled *Quantum Mechanics* by Leonard Susskind, a quantum physicist and teacher. He noted several times in his text that the quantum realm is counterintuitive, cannot be understood through our normal senses, and requires a relatively high level understanding of mathematics to be able to start to comprehend its existence. I respectfully disagree.

Certainly the minutia of the internal specifics of quantum mechanics require mathematics and technology to confirm experimentally. Just as in depth understanding of the micro level of human cells and their biochemistry and physiology require a high level of training in the relevant sciences and the technology to back it up. But it is also relevant and possible to understand the deeper processes and systems of the body, and of the cosmos, through a more wholistic and unified view. This approach does not require the high level math and science, yet can still discover fundamental principles and connections in the quantum realm and human health. This is qi training and practice.

CHAPTER 2 - EDUCATION

Let's return for a moment to Jill Bolte Taylor's realization regarding the activities of the left and right hemisphere's of her brain. After her stroke it took Jill 8 years to recover from the damage done to the left side of her brain. But in that time it is also clear that she became fluid at moving her focus from the right to the left, or the left to the right hemispheres. She suggested we could choose the hemisphere we want to act from during our daily activities. Her capacity to make these shifts is not usual for most humans, and she did not provide any specific advice or techniques at the time for facilitating others to gain this skill. The very unfortunate occurrence in her personal history of having a stroke had this unexpected positive outcome of providing her with the capacity to enter fully into her right brain connectivity with the energetic fields. But how are we to accomplish this same adeptness at switching brain hemispheres?

In addition, let's think about where she is actually going when she fully engages the right sided brain experience. As she described it, this is a universe of no individuality, physical form, or personal history. She provides a view of a cosmic expanse of energy that is infinite and engendering an experience of deep well being. This expansive/contractive self with no physical boundaries is coupled with her very personal and individualized self that recalls her specific personal history, professional training and activities, and has all the qualities we usually associate with an autonomous human being situated in time recalling the past while planning for the future.

If we look at her descriptions of these two realities of her experience, what they imply is that on one hand her left brain is primarily living in this physical world that on a macro level provides us with the reality that we, and generations of those before us, have considered to be the mainstay of our daily existence. And on the other hand, her description of the reality of vortexes of energy and barrierless sensations of connectivity with everything in the universe implies an experiential access to the quantum realm, a realm that has been discovered and researched in science only in the last century or so. How could this be?

The simplest explanation for this is that the evolution of our brains, and the rest of our bodies, has been going on over millennium refining our awareness and relationship with the external physical world we must survive in as humans, and also with our connectivity to the quantum realm and the vibrational ocean of energy that is fundamental to who we are back into the eons of time. And of course, from the ground up we are binaries - particulate and formless - as noted in quantum mechanics and ancient Asian thought.

And why wouldn't that be the case? It makes sense that if the Quantum / Newtonian binary has been in place for millions of years in our universe, that the evolution of forms in this milieu would have connection to and awareness of both aspects of the whole. It is only recently in the history of evolution that human civilization, particularly western technological societies, has emphasized the autonomous individual and the attributes associated with left brain activities. This programming and practice could have stunted or blocked access to our right brain capacity to live fully in the moment, and our capacity for awareness of the aspect of our self that is interconnected with the rest of our universe.

In our present culture this kind of natural cosmic experience of self is often thought to occur, if at all, with exceptional spiritual experiences and/or drug induced states. Its subjective sensations are not trusted by any objective science leaning intelligentsia, and there is little to no training available in the west to support rigorous right brain development in this arena. If anything such training is suppressed and we are left with a muted capacity to sense the quantum realm to such a degree that our scientists state that it is impossible, without having a high level of mathematical understanding. In other words, it is only through the professional authority and acumen of the trained scientist that we can expect to have any knowledge of our own strange quantum reality. Yet probably, if you've ever seen Australian aboriginal artwork, you could reasonably infer that from its imagery they are more directly connected and aware of this realm than their scientific counterparts.

I suggest qi gong training, and other practices

of largely non-technological societies, provide strengthening of so-called right brain activity and its access to the experiential aspect of our shared quantum reality. For in deep internal qi gong training it is common place to experience versions of what Jill Bolte Taylor described. If the fundamental Qi activity of expansion and contraction is practiced regularly, it directly engages the kinesthetic/energetic aspect of our right brain activity and body, that is an access point to having experiences of our self as connectivity. Qi activity is for most humans most easily accessible internally through awareness of breathing, the binary of inhalation/exhalation, expansion/contraction, coming and going; and externally through a variety of body movements that accentuate and share these same expansive/ contractive qualities. A wide range of spiritual and self-discovery disciplines point to breath awareness and full body engagement as a critical component to promote more sensitivity and awareness of the larger expanse of our being.

Our programmed distrust of this side of ourselves has led to a culture based on the primacy of individuality, and with that belief comes a wide range of illnesses that could be described simply at their core as being manifestations of separation anxiety. Thus our lack of feeling grounded and connected to our universe. This generates symptoms of distrust, paranoia, anxiety, unbridled desires and ambitions, and doubts/rigidity regarding our role in life; that harm both ourselves and our environment. To regain balance and harmony we need to regain a trust in our intuitive/connected self. From this foundation, with regularly practiced methods that connect us with the right side of our brain and our whole body, we discover the energetic sea that quantum physics and Chinese medicine both state we are part of.

From this viewpoint, the balanced scientist or

physician would have a different approach to education than is presently offered in order to prepare them for inquiry into, and engagement with, the whole of health or the cosmos. This balanced training program for professionals would have rigorous training in analytical and rational thinking for developing intellectual knowledge and objective reasoning. It would also have rigorous instruction and practice in mind/body integration techniques that utilize awareness of the present moment and our connection with the earth and our environment to provide improved sensitivity and openness to the wisdom of this immediate universe we are embedded in and connected to. In other words adequate instruction to enhance both left and right brain approaches to experiencing reality.

But Qi training does not stop at that point. The nature of binaries is that the balanced awareness of the whole comes from being able to incorporate both aspects *simultaneously* into the engagement with whatever endeavor is occurring. In other words, it is not enough to choose left or right, it is also vital to discover and practice how these two seemingly oppositional aspects integrate and merge to form our whole self, and perform the functions and efforts of our daily lives. Since Qi is a term describing the whole of these activities, both the limited expanding/contracting particular being and the cosmic infinitely expanding/contracting being, it is necessary to find the place where these two "selves" meet. This is recognized as the transformative axis of Qi in which "many become one, and one becomes many".

To give a practical example, in acupuncture training it is common to train students to be knowledgable regarding relevant medical theory and its application to diagnosis and clinical reasoning, and thus to the generation and analysis of treatment plans. This is standard rational medicine, the structure of this process being very similar to the elements of clinical reasoning in biomedicine. The other aspect of acupuncture training can be to provide for an embodied stillness that assists the student in directly feeling the rhythms and shifts of energy in the body of the patient, where obstruction or depletion of the flows and rhythms could exist. This activity requires an opposite skill set; an ability to suspend rational thought, focusing attention on the moment and the sensations and flows that arise when this connected awareness is tapped in to. It is in this state that practitioners and patients may both sense more "connectivity", that is Qi. Then, by integrating these two sources of knowledge and information (from left and right), the practitioner student is expected to formulate an intention for treatment that is manifested through direct physical engagement with the patient with techniques such as acupuncture, moxibustion and massage. It is here that the integrated approach of rational intent and unified connectivity are brought together to provide a treatment experience that, if it accesses that place of balance and integration, is transformative.

One form of instruction to assist the access to the "quantum self", the field aspect of your personal particle/wave binary is to use what I call "embodied imagination". As Einstein noted: "Imagination is more important than knowledge. For knowledge is limited to all we now know and understand,, whereas imagination embraces the entire world and all there ever will be to know and understand."

To illustrate this form of training, I will end this chapter with a simple version of an exercise that is part of what is called Qi Gong, or qi practice; and with it utilize this embodied imagination to amplify the results of the practice. Daily practice of this in the morning and evening, and any other time you have a bit of space and time, will gradually deepen your capacity for experiencing the quantum side of your self, and the connectivity that is associated with it. As this occurs you will also begin to naturally discover ways to continue deepening your practice. It is as if your deeper self wants you to return to this more expanded awareness and provides the insights to assist you along the way.

QI EXERCISE #1

Find a quiet place. (Actually this ancient instruction that is found at the beginning of many texts on yoga, meditation and qi gong is really pointing at you finding the quiet place within yourself, as well as externally, before you start the practice.)

For this exercise we will stand up and do a simple stretching movement. It can also be practiced in a sitting position. First, pay attention to whatever sensation you feel where your feet meet the floor/ground. Take a few moments to sense and stay with this experience. When you feel ready, imagine you feel a sensation of inhaling through the soles of your feet as your lungs inhale, and then a sensation of exhaling through the soles of your feet as you exhale. Do this for at least five slow breaths. (Over time as you practice this you can extend the intention to imagining that with the inhale you draw the energy up from the soles of your feet to your lower abdomen; and with the exhale, that the flow travels from your abdomen back down to the ground. But in the beginning it is most important to simply establish the sensation of feeling the inhale/exhale in the soles of your feet.)

After doing a few of these breaths with the inhale/exhale sensation in your soles, with your next inhale slowly raise your arms up over your head like they are wings until they are stretched vertically over your head. *Keep your awareness of breathing in your feet as you do this*, with the inhale matching the length of time it takes to extend your arms above your head. Pause. Then, as you slowly exhale have your arms swing down like wings to your sides as you also imagine flow going down into your feet and into the earth. Do this stretch with breathing at least five more times......

When you feel ready you could now also start an embodied exercise imagining you are a tree (or a flower) moving through the four seasons. With the beginning of your inhale it is spring and the sap and the energy of the earth are rising lifting your limbs up to the sky and sun. With the full extension of your arms above with the full inhale you enter summer and a space where you are stretching and open to the sun and heavens and the radiation of energy down from above (while rooted to the earth through your awareness in your feet). Hold this space for a few beats. Then as you exhale and the arms descend, imagine autumn and the descending energy of the tree returning to the roots in the earth or to form a seed. With full exhale feel the sense of connection with the earth and the quiet of that foundation in winter. Hold this for a few moments. Then begin your next inhalation and your next cycle of life and death as you breathe through the four seasons of growth and decay. Do this for at least five cycles.

When you finish, place your hands on your lower belly as if embracing yourself there and slowly breath into that space five times......

Another addition to this exercise would be to do it while also standing in front of and looking at one of your favorite trees.   Trees are great instructors in this regard :) If the idea of learning from, or breathing with trees seems silly to you, then trust me - this is simply your limited self supplying you with the thought due to being afraid of letting go of its dominance.

There are several levels of embodied imagination in this exercise. Please do what is comfortable for you and take your time, while keeping your breathing relaxed. It is normal to have a few strange sensations as you begin this if you have never done any simple rhythmic breathing stretches. I recommend you particularly keep your awareness in the soles of your feet as much as you can as you go through all the aspects of this practice.

Being aware of the sensation in the soles of your feet is not a bad meditative device to do on a regular basis through the day. It has been recommended in textual materials by health providers and Qi practitioners in Asia going back over three thousand years, and remains a valuable practice in contemporary times. Essentially, putting your awareness in your feet draws your mental awareness down and embeds your mind/spirit more in your body. This balances our societal tendencies of having multiple activities that put us, or keep us "in our head" a lot. Practicing grounding can by itself have profound effects on blood pressure, upper body muscle tension, headaches, anxiety and the like...

CHAPTER 3 - TRANSFORMATION

Throughout most of modern history we have gotten by believing we exist in space; this space being an absolutely huge phenomena separate from us; and time, that is also some absolutely infinite universally measured ticking. Einstein sort of punctured that balloon in the early 1900's, but it does not seem that his profound and more accurate realizations have made a lot of impact on the way most folks view their experience in the universe. That's reasonable given in our perceived, though ultimately illusory physical world, Newton's assertions regarding the nature of absolute space and absolute time appear to hold up just fine.

But once we enter the quantum side of everything things just aren't the same. Essentially, what Einstein proved mathematically is that space and time are not separate, but are in fact another, and one of the grandest binaries in the universe. We exist in spacetime. They are intimately intertwined with the same dynamic that we referred to in the previous chapter regarding quantum binaries. In addition since there are no absolute landmarks or measurements in this spacetime configuration, everything immersed in it has its own relative spacetime. That is, your spacetime and my spacetime, though they may seem to be the same, are actually unique and specific to each of us. This is a fundamental finding of the theory of relativity. Probably one of the most accessible places to read about this in more depth is in Walter Isaacson's biography of Albert entitled *Einstein: His Life and Universe*. Chapters 5, 6, 7 & 9 go into detail about Albert's life and times when he had these epiphanies and the thought processes that went along with them.

Specifically, in Chapter 7 in a subsection entitled "The Equivalence of Gravity and Acceleration" we read of Einstein's self described "happiest thought in my life", which was also the origin of his developing his general theory of relativity, that space and time were not absolutes, but conjoined in a "relative" space-time. This first "thought" was the imagined experience that "if a person falls freely, he will not feel his own weight". This then led to identifying that the experience of acceleration and gravity were identical, and thus one could not ever tell if one is moving or stationary since there are no fixed landmarks to go by. So the theory of relativity and spacetime did not originate from high level math or technological findings, but simply from the embodied kinesthetic experience of freely falling bodies, acceleration, and gravity - accessing right brain sensibilities - that is - Qi.

For us in this little book you are now reading,

the hope is that Einstein's realization will assist us to imagine what it feels like, to know we live in the center of our own personal spacetime cosmos. That at your core you are the author of your space and time. They are not absolute fixed identities separate from you. They are intimately part of you. So as you move through the world your spacetime moves with you. In fact, though it is so tiny as to be immeasurable in normal circumstances, when you move in your space it slows down your time. So, taking an impossible example, if you flew in a space ship at close to the speed of light for a decade or so and then returned to my doorstep, and we both had atomic watches on our wrists the whole time, a comparison of our clocks would show I had aged more than you (a few minutes perhaps).

Now this may not seem that important on a daily basis. Just like when Brian Green, a physicist who also does a lot of writing for the public on quantum matters suggested that from a quantum perspective the location of the origin of the universe, the Big Bang, is inside each of us. That realization also does not necessarily have much impact on how we approach our mundane daily activities. But both of them can have a powerful impact on how we experience ourself in our Qi universe. Quantum science speaking, you are the center of your space-time, you are the origin of your universe.

When we are fixated in our particular indi-vidualized self, a polar aspect of our "binary being", we are unable to sense or understand the "other" side, the "la la land". It is actu-ally invisible to us according to both quantum and Asian theory. Thus the findings described above may feel counterintuitive to you at this moment since the capacity to read this book implies you are presently at least somewhat fixed in your individual self. But if you slip into the side of yourself where you experience yourself as the ocean of existence, then the epiphanies of Einstein have a profound effect on your experience of the world and your place in it as an individual. Your Qi gong will transform.

For me, the above experience of Einstein and the direct personal experience in Qi gong demonstrate how practice/experience can inform/transform science/knowledge, and how science/knowledge can inform/transform practice. By that I mean the interdependence of your "knowledge" self and your "experiential" self in learning and transformation. Regarding Einstein's epiphany about the relativity of time and space, his experience informed his creation of a theoretical framework, and in turn this insight could make a significant difference in your experience in Qi practice. To do this though you have to have a Qi practice. Then you take the Einstein spacetime realization and engage it within your practice.

The integration of these two is what leads to transformation.

I have colleagues in Qi practice who resist strongly bringing any contemporary understanding of our universe into their approach and understanding to Qi. Particularly the physics of it. And I have friends in academia and science that rebel at any suggestion that their subjective experience could be useful in aiding their scientific inquiry. To me both sides of this dynamic reflect the finding in Neils Bohr's complementarity discovery, the more you fixate on one side of the whole - the more you cannot see or understand the other side, and hence the whole itself.

I invite you to take every counterintuitive finding in quantum physics that you can find, and plug them into whatever level of meditative or yogic or Qi practice you have, and see what that simultaneous holding of both sides of your self engenders in your experiential practice. Then take whatever transformative event occurs from that union, and bring it back to your "thinking" self, and see again how that transforms your view of the world and your role in it. It is this back and forth from yin to yang and yang to yin and the meeting of the two that Chinese thought, and quantum physics, state generate existence. You are now participating in that emergence.

CHAPTER 4 - ZERO

I think it is time we face the grandmama of all koans. Koans, if you are unfamiliar with them, are educational devices developed within Zen training programs to assist students to cross over from their rational thinking / problem solving mind to their formless boundary-less side of themselves, and back again. To do this the teacher provides the student with a quasi-riddle, one that could not be answered by reasoning, thinking, rationality - but instead requires demonstrating the leap to being able to connect with and manifest the understanding that emerges from the connectivity side of yourself, you as Qi. To do this students will often first make great efforts with their thinking mind to solve the matter through objectifying the riddle because this is often the only way they know to solve problems. The outcome of this effort is often effectively exhausting that thinking faculty. This is one way that can then allow the right side of the brain, and the spontaneous "field" side of you to emerge more clearly. And from that perspective immediately appears your personal solution, your insight into the problem. An awakening.

Zen teachers are called Zen masters, partially because they have demonstrated to their teachers they can move fluidly between the two aspects of themselves, as well as integrate them. And also because they have demonstrated they are capable of recognizing when their students are able to make this leap and assist them with the self discovery process. Instructional style in present times is then a methodology providing koans or pointers to encourage the student's personal effort to discover how to bridge the gap between the linear self and the cosmic side, and then when this is demonstrated to recognize and confirm this shift. Often this process takes many years, and now there are in some schools of practice defined stages to this development.

Going back into the history of China, where these instructional techniques first started to emerge (over a thousand years ago), you can find story after story of the provocative encounters between teacher and student as they struggled together to break open the student's fixation on individuality. The struggles and stories from these early practitioners who did both physical qi gong exercises and meditative inquiry into the nature of their reality, are mind boggling and enlightening.

Discovering something that cannot be explained by our rational thought and our science to date, but is still demonstrated to exist, is a case of a modern day koan. And quantum physics offers a plethora of these examples.

The granddaddy of them being the so-called entanglement of particles.

Take two particles that are suitably inter-twined and send one of them billions of light years away to a galaxy far far away. Interact with either one of these particles. Instantaneously, that is simultaneously, the two particles act together in response to your inter-action. The speed of light, and therefore what we assume is the fastest mode of communica-tion possible, would take billions of light years of time to communicate from one particle to the other. But in fact, they interact as if they are one - no communication as such occurs - no separation, no time, no space. It defies modern scientific understanding of space and time. Essentially this entanglement demon-strates that somewhere, somehow, somewhen in this reality we are part of; there is a place, a way, a dimension that has no space and no time. That spacetime simply does not apply.

Einstein hated this finding until the day he died. Ironically he developed the math that first predicted this non-local activity, this "spooky action at a distance", this union that defied the speed of light and every other aspect of our known universe. He could not get it. How is it possible to have two photons separated by a trillion light years still react simultaneously when you stimulate one of the photons, when the fundamental law of the quantum and physical universe is that nothing can travel faster than the speed of light? These entangled particles defied Einstein. They act as one. They are as one? How can this be?

As often with these discoveries of things we cannot comprehend, that has not stopped future generations of scientists and inventors from trying to find ways to take this discovery and develop practical applications that will either make money, or provide the owner with the capacity for world domination, or both.

This is true with entanglement as well. The Chinese, the Americans, and others, are developing entanglement computers that allow communication instantly across any distance with no ability for anyone to interfere, tap into, or decode that communication, because there is no transmission of anything in entanglement. A military and high tech bonanza. But still, no one can explain how this activity is possible.

Therefore, if you can put on your "the universe is a wonder; an awe-inspiring, mystery-type-place cap" and contemplate this no space, no time dimension. How do you answer this? Returning to my suggestion in the last chapter, quantum physics can inform qi practice, and qi practice can inform quantum physics. Take this no space / no time dimension and see if you can find it in your qi gong, your meditations, your experience of qi.

As a koan, entanglement, provides the same

question as its old Chinese counterparts. In fact, one of the most famous koans of ancient times sounds eerily like the description of entanglement. In this koan the student is faced with understanding and experiencing "Mu" (Japanese) - "Wu" (Chinese). The meaning in English is approximately the Void, Emptiness, Nothingness, or simply "No". Now, up until recently in the west Void meant emptiness, as in there is nothing there - a vacuum - just like outer space. But with quantum physics it is now understood that this Void of outer space is actually anything but a vacuum, it is full of interconnected vibrating energy.

This is also the case with ancient understanding of the Void, at least by the masters. Though it may be that the students then also held a belief that Emptiness was completely empty, and not filled with vibrational force, with Qi. So the effort of the student was to discover the "No" , the vibrating "No", that knew no boundaries, including no space and no time. The barrier that is no barrier. And the commentary explains that when realized the student will be holding hands with all the teachers back into the eons of time. And this, I suspect, was not fanciful writing, this was the true expectation of the outcome of this research. The student would transcend space and time and hold hands with everybody. Up until recently that would have seemed metaphorical, but how can you now explain the technologically proven "Entanglement"? Is that a metaphor too?

So I suggest again, quantum physics has gifted us with this mystery regarding the underlying nature of reality, a place where time and space as we know it do not exist, and it therefore stands as the grandest of all koans to date.

When you do qi practice, qi gong, you do movements that engage your breath and spirit and body in expanding and contracting movements. And if you can; imagining them as infinitely expanding and infinitely contracting. They amount to an all embracing cosmic hug. All existence of any kind in any place in the cosmos manifests this simple but mysterious activity constantly. Why expand and contract? There is no fixation or freezing of this activity.

Even though our linear mind may arrange, for example, a visual of our physical reality that it is limited and looks fixed, the real fact is that it is an electromagnetic matrix that holds together what we call matter, and it is that force that repels us when we "hit" something physical, it is not that we actually hit or touch something. The force repels us without any actual physical contact.

This reality generally does not agree with the understanding we have of our sensory inputs of physical objects. But by participating in the fundamental activity of Qi consciously, you can tap into the sensation of this reality where everything is energy, including that the ground beneath your feet is not physical substance but an abyss of infinite energetic vibrations. And once you begin to explore this expanding/contracting reality you may also begin to resonate with this dimension of no time / no space. A hug where time doesn't exist.

To repeat again, your brain and every cell of your body is wired, and has been wired for millennium, down through the generations, to access the reality of being a contractive/expansive force. This Qi activity is your being. You are both an imperfect limited individual / citizen of this planet, and a universal force that is infinitely contracting/expanding. You do have within you the capacity to be in a timeless no space state. To directly experience what quantum physicists call entanglement.

And just briefly, the very naming by physicists

of this experience as being "entanglement" indicates a left brain perspective. Entangled implies at least two somethings somehow mixed or tied together. But this experience is not about two. In fact, it is likely maybe not best described as being about one. This dimension of no time no space no boundary within you might be most accurately described in English as zero. Nada.

QI EXERCISE #2

Here is an exercise to assist this discovery process. The initial paragraphs will be a description of instruction, slightly modified, but given for hundreds of years in Asia regarding correct posture and positioning for internal qi gong or meditative practice. I suggest you do Exercise #1 as a warm-up prior to doing this. You may want to record this for yourself, edited if you like, so you can initially listen to the instructions while getting into the meditation - a guided meditation if you will. With time these steps will come naturally to you and can be practiced in whatever venue you find yourself where you are sitting (or standing).

First, find a quiet place. We will do this in a seated position, though standing qi gong is also fine. Choose whatever sitting position feels right to you. It may be contemporary western style sitting in a chair with your feet flat on the floor, or sitting in a cross legged fashion as is favored by meditators influenced by Asian practices. If you use a cross legged approach, please insure you are sitting so that your spine is erect and your knees are also connecting to the ground. That is, you will likely use a cushion under you to get into this position. Once comfortably seated, bring your awareness to everywhere in your body where you connect with the floor, or chair, or cushion. Stay with that sensation for awhile allowing your mind to settle into that awareness and feeling the sensations in your whole body, but particularly with where you interface with what is holding you up.

Keeping your spine erect and posture in alignment, slightly tilt forward and backward and left and right to locate the position where you feel most centered over your personal center of gravity, like the trunk of a tree. Anchor your awareness by imagining at the base of your spine you are holding hands with a friend. This will help to further settle and embed your mind in your body. Check that your chest is uplifted slightly so your breathing is open and your chin is slightly tucked so that your neck and head are in better alignment with your spine. Imagine a cord connected to the vertex of your head gently drawing upward. It is important to keep your back erect and your posture relaxed but in alignment with gravity. Insure your jaw is not tense and your tongue tip is connected to the roof of your mouth. Check your shoulder blades that they are slightly drawn together to counteract the hunching forward we often do with computers and books and the like. Take a few minutes to keep checking these pointers for body posture so that you begin to feel comfortable with this positioning. Like a tree rooted to the earth as well as opening up to the sun.

Become aware of your breathing. You may want to briefly do the raising and lowering of your arms with the breath cycle as we did in Qi exercise #1 in Chapter 2 in order to remind your body of fully breathing. Fully inhale - pause - fully exhale - pause, and continue; sensing this breathing experience as your WHOLE being, with every physical and mental aspect of you inhaling and exhaling together - your nose, your toes, the tips of your hair, your skin, your mind - they all expand and contract. Gently observe if you experience the feeling of simultaneous expansion/contraction as you breathe in and out.

In any case be gentle with yourself and stay grounded by keeping awareness of the sensation in the parts of your body where you are connected with the floor/ground.

Begin to imagine that interface of connection

with the earth also joining breathing so you and the earth are simply a breathing process. Stay with this activity for a few minutes. With time and practice it will get easier and easier and deeper and deeper.

For your hand posture for this exercise I'm going to ask you to simply hold your hands together, again imagining like you are holding hands with a good friend or family member you trust or care for, and hold them just under your navel. As you inhale feel the movement up your spine and as you exhale feel the movement flowing down your arms, into your hands, and then connecting in your lower belly. Do this for a bit to see if you can get into a cozy connected feeling in your belly and hands.

Again, with time and practice, slowly, slowly putting all this together will create a settled and poised state.

The sitting instructions provided above assist you in moving more and more into the "right" side of your brain and this experience of feeling more flow or connectivity or peacefulness. We are now ready to begin the next part of a further "embodied imagination" practice. I suggest you start with a lighted candle in a darkened room or a favorite star in the night sky. Other possibilities are a favorite tree or flower.

After taking several minutes to settle in a bit, turn your awareness to a lighted candle or star. As you gaze at the star please also gaze within yourself to see if there is a place that resonates with the light you see externally. To assist this, imagine the candle or star is also breathing with you, that you are inhaling/exhaling together. Keep with this for a bit, feeling open, but aware, breathing with your full body, your connection with the earth, and the light. Whereever you can sense this connection will help you learn of the relationship you have between your "inner" and "outer" worlds.

Allow yourself several minutes with this activity, continuing to maintain postural alignment, friendship feeling in your hands and the base of your spine, and full body breathing. If after several minutes this candle/star engagement exercise is providing no sense of a link between you and the light, then simply let go of that intention and remain in the sitting, breathing, grounded state for awhile feeling whatever comes up and letting it pass away. This practice took me years so you may not reap instantaneous results :) Maintain your awareness of the physical sensation connecting with the floor. About 15 minutes in the beginning of practice is a good amount of time for this meditative qi gong. As you practice more, you can extend the amount of time, but I don't suggest going beyond a half hour.

The sitting qi gong practice described here is

first to help quiet your being and bring mind, breath and body together. The awareness on breathing and awareness of the connection to the earth help to settle and encourage flow. The step of seeking resonance with a star in the night sky or a candle is to find where in you there is this accord, like when you sing with another person and hit the same note. It has that same spirit to it. So it is not completely active or passive on your part, it is an engagement in relationship that requires both "listening" and connecting, to hit the right chord together. You are seeing if you can do this with the star.

As you and the star breathe, you share the beat of the heart of life together. You are also both surrounded by the abyss of space that shares in this breathing activity. Feel the great silence of space with the great light of the star as they engage and support each other.

As you practice this activity more, possibly

finding within you some resonance with the external "object", I suggest specifically you explore if there is a resonance in your lower abdomen that feels an affinity with the candle or star. Gaze inward feeling the sensations in your lower belly as you also look outward at the light with your mutual breathing. This connection will be helpful in further Qi gong practice.

CHAPTER 5 - COME HEALING

In the last chapter I introduced you to the star in the night sky or the candle in the darkened room as your teacher. By listening inside yourself as you engage this light and dark, you are seeking to find your place of resonance with their vibration. You are learning from them and the further you go with this, the more you will find they have something to teach you. Remember Einstein's quote regarding the power of imagination. Embodied imagination provides the capacity for deeper understanding of your self and your relationship with the universe.

In this chapter I want to have you consider the reverse approach to Qi practice. As this little book has noted often, existence is binaries. Thus the need to include both sides to better understand the whole, and then someday to be able to sit with both simultaneously.

I recall a little book I read several decades ago called the *Kinship with All Life*, by J. Allen Boone. The first section was a description of one man's efforts to communicate with a dog that he was tasked with babysitting. Apparently this was not just any dog, it was actually the most famous dog actor in the movies at that time, named Strongheart. A German shepherd, the dog was exceptionally intelligent and responsive to the people he was involved with. As the man spent time with the dog he had glimpses of experiences where the dog seemed to know what the man wanted or where he was going, possibly before he did. He began to realize that the dog could understand him profoundly more deeply than he could understand the dog. So he took on the task of attempting to communicate with the dog.

This was a trial and error sort of effort, with a lot of error in the beginning. You can pick up the little book if you are interested in his journey. I will move to where he finally, somewhat accidentally, discovered how he could engage and communicate/commune with the dog. What he discovered was that what was most important was to bring his best spirit, his best intention, his best openness, to the moment and the relationship. The two of them would often go to a ridge overlooking the city and there they would sit and he would work on this practice. What is it to bring your best intention, best spirit to the moment? How does that look or feel? What do you think about, or not think about?

It is actually not necessarily so easy to discover a fully embodied "bestness" of who you are in this present moment in relationship with anyone. But that is what we will explore in this chapter.

Why? Because it appears that discovering in yourself the best kind of stance and intention you have in the moment puts you in the zone where you discover your connectivity and relationship with the whole.

First, let me sidestep to a growing area of research in the west. In 1952, a physicist named Winfried Otto Schumann mathematically predicted that there is an all pervading and constant deluge of vibrational energy within our earth's atmosphere generated by lightning. Lightning strikes around the planet about 8 million times a day generating a particular set of frequencies that then are present in our atmosphere at all times and therefore are being absorbed by everything on this planet. And this has been going on for millions of years. Now called the Schumann Resonance, these vibrations are in the ELF range, that is Extremely Low Frequency vibrations from about 5 Hz to 50 Hz with the primary frequency being 7.8 Hz. This resonance can be measured everywhere on our planet's surface and resonates within the space between the ionosphere and the earth's surface.

Since the discovery of the Schumann Resonance finer tuned equipment, most notably the SQUID that measures the bioelectromagnetic radiations from living beings, have shown that these frequencies are within and emitted by living beings on the planet. In humans, they have recorded these frequencies radiating more strongly from particular organs, the heart and brain having the strongest biomagnetic signal in most people. The exception seems to be some bodywork or healer practitioners that have a stronger signal emanating from their hands at a more significant strength than the normal radiations measured from the heart and other parts of the body. Essentially though, every cell of a human vibrates at these frequencies. These emanations match the frequency range of the planetary vibrations (For more on this please see the references section for *Energy Medicine: The Scientific Basis*, by Oschman.)

Additional health research, primarily done in Russia for the last 100 years and only recently in the West, shows that these ELF frequencies, when applied to injured tissues have a healing effect on those tissues. The frequency used in treatment is tissue specific. This is based on Einstein's initial discovery that frequency, not signal strength, increases the strength of vibrating photons. That is to strengthen "blue" photons you need more blue frequency, not simply stronger light that isn't blue frequency. Therefore it was found that the frequencies for bone regeneration for example, are different from those for the skin or for muscles, etc.. In essence, an appropriate healthy frequency focused on an area of injury that exhibits a disrupted frequency, will amplify the "healthy" frequencies in the tissues and encourage the speed of recovery.

This approach to healing is also being explored with internal conditions like cancer, to assist both in early diagnosis and treatment. Russians have used this medical therapy for decades in the treatment of dysfunction, particularly in athletes. They have developed diagnostic equipment to assess disharmonies in frequencies, as well as equipment that mimics the body's healthy frequencies and is used in treatment. Since this frequency based medicine is not one that the pharmaceutical industry can use to develop products and make money, there has been little funding in the west approved to research this ELF phenomena, and until recently findings in this vibrational approach to therapy were suppressed and ridiculed (Well, in some circles they are still being ridiculed).

What has also been discovered is that some

healers that use their hands, either directly touching the body, or off the body, generate these same ELF signals when working on patients. It is hypothesized that these frequencies from human hands adjust to the frequency range associated with the ELF needed by the area of injury on the patient the practitioner is working on. In other words, like lightning, which is drawn to strike certain energetic anomalies on the earth's surface, the human hand may also be drawn to adjust its radiation to the dynamics of the tissue being treated. Given the millions of years humans have been evolving on this planet and mothers and healers have been working with their hands with the intention to heal injuries in the young or the infirm, it is possible there has been evolutionary development of this vibrational capacity. In East Asian Medicine we call this feeling or sensing the Qi and healing with Qi.

In the last couple of decades a paradigm based on quantum field theory has developed that may hold promise for research in the future. It utilizes the model of a "biofield" to explain the connectivity of individuals, even at a distance. See the reference section of this text for a journal issue of *Global Advances in Health* that is dedicated to articles on this topic. This field approach recognizes how we are both particulate physical beings and fields of energy and that this understanding could be used in developing diagnostic and treatment strategies based on this connectivity. This perspective is also being used to explain the efficacy of modalities in East Asian medicine as well as other natural therapies from around the planet. It indicates there could be a much less invasive and less toxic approach to therapy developed in biomedicine then is presently available.

The history in less technological cultures on our planet to harmonize the biofield / individual dynamic, that is to improve Qi harmony or vibrational wellbeing, includes a range of practices to enhance the healer/patient relationship. Examples include ritual, meditative practices, qi gong, yoga, prayer, music, drumming, dance, chanting, mind altering drugs, visualizations, and mantras, to name a few. Quantum physics now demonstrates that everything; be it called a virus, an evil spirit, a damaged tissue, an obsessive thought, an emotional trauma, an organ malfunction, or a toxic chemical; all are fundamentally vibrational expanding/contracting energy, that is Qi. Thus ancient cultures who sensed this cosmic reality directly through their own versions of Qi practices developed treatment methods that were also vibrational in their therapeutic approach.

These vibrational states can be differentiated at a basic level by the frequency of their contractive/expansive activity. This knowledge can be used for diagnosis and treatment. The quantum medicine of the future will likely evolve out of present day practices that use anomalies of body frequencies to do early diagnosis of health conditions, as well as present day research in how appropriate frequencies amplify healthy frequencies in the body to stimulate restoration. It could also include therapies that use frequencies that are keyed to destroy pathogens while being harmless to healthy tissue. Maybe it will be called Qi medicine...

The point of this information showing up here is to highlight that the natural healthy biomagnetic radiations of your body are also beneficial to the world surrounding your body. You, simply standing there, are radiating healing energy all around you - by doing nothing. The more you resonate with the earth's vibrations, the more your body radiates these signals. This natural state of resonance with the earth's frequencies quiets your "mind of separation". Your qi gong strengthens this connection. Or as Leonard Cohen puts it in his song Anthem:

> Ring the bell that still can ring
> Forget your perfect offering
> There is a crack, a crack in everything
> That's how the light gets in.

Thus, the definition of the "better" you is the natural you, the you that is simply accepting of who you truly are. Regardless of any concerns you have of your physical or mental disarray, your imperfectness, your past mistakes, you are naturally manifesting a grounded state that vibrationally resonates with your world. As Taoists would say, your qi activity, that is the true you, and the nature activity are the same. They are with the Tao. You are the Tao. And thus, when you settle into it, this "best" arrives as a formless universal connectivity that cultivates your particulate self to form a relationship with the whole.

QI EXERCISE #3

There are exercises that can help you manifest more completely your natural state. Below is one of them used to assist individuals interested in healing.

This exercise is complementary to Exercise #2. Both #2 and #3 utilize Exercise #1 as their base. From that grounding you can practice being the receiver or the provider. By practicing both you will find with time their relationship. That as it is stated in yin/yang theory; the yin in its final phase will transform into and nourish the yang, and the yang will in its final phase in turn transform and support yin. Thus they engender each other - simultaneously. To personally clarify and experience this activity that you are already participating in, practice the exercise provided below, alternating it with practicing Exercise #2.

We will do this exercise sitting, though again, it can be done just as well in a standing position. As before, follow the instructions given in the first few paragraphs of Exercise #2. I will repeat them here. After that this exercise will explore a different embodied imagination activity.

First, find a quiet place. We will do this in a seated position though this is not required. Choose whatever sitting position feels right to you. It may be contemporary western style sitting in a chair with your feet flat on the floor, or sitting in a cross legged fashion as is favored by meditators influenced by Asian practices. Once seated, bring your awareness to everywhere in your body where you connect with the floor, or chair, or cushion. Stay with that sensation for awhile allowing your mind to settle into that awareness and feeling the sensations in your whole body, but particularly with where you interface with what is holding you up. Keeping your spine erect and posture in alignment, slightly tilt forward and backward and left and right to locate the position where you feel most centered over your personal center of gravity, like the trunk of a tree.

Anchor your awareness by imagining at the base of your spine you are holding hands with a friend. Check that your chest is uplifted slightly so your breathing is open and your chin is slightly tucked so that your neck and head are in better alignment with your spine. Imagine a cord connected to the vertex of your head gently drawing upward. It is important to keep your back erect and your posture relaxed but in alignment with gravity. Insure your jaw is not tense and your tongue tip is connected to the roof of your mouth. Check your shoulder blades that they are slightly drawn together to counteract the hunching forward we often do with computers and books and the like. Take a few minutes to keep checking these pointers for body posture so that you begin to feel comfortable with this positioning.

Become aware of your breathing. You may want to briefly do the raising and lowering of your arms with the breath cycle as we did in the earlier Qi Exercise #1 in Chapter 2 in order to remind your body of fully breathing. Inhale gently and fully - pause - exhale gently and fully - pause - and continue. This breathing experience is with your WHOLE being, every cell inhales and exhales together, your nose, your toes, the tips of your hair, your skin, your mind - they all expand and contract. Gently observe if you experience the feeling of simultaneous expansion/contraction as you breathe.

In any case be gentle with yourself and stay grounded by keeping awareness of the sensation in the parts of your body where you are connected with the floor/ground.

Begin to imagine that interface of connection with the earth also joining breathing so you and the earth are simply a breathing process. Stay with this activity for a few minutes. With time and practice it will get easier and easier and deeper and deeper.

For the hand position of this qi gong we will hold our hands so that your forearms are parallel with the floor and your palms facing each other separated by the same distance as the width of your body. With inhalation imagine the qi moving up your spine from your lower belly and then as you exhale flowing down your arms and into your hands. Follow this flow for several breaths.

Now we will imagine that Planet Earth is small enough to fit between your hands and is slowly revolving in space. Allow your breath and energy to now flow from your hands into this revolving globe. This is your earth, facing whatever troubles you want to consider at this point. Therefore now bring your intention for its support to your hands and transmit to the planet itself. For several minutes practice the circulation of energy, starting from your lower abdomen, inhaling up to your shoulders, exhaling down your arms, into your hands, and into the planet - integrated with your intention for the planet and its well-being. Check in with your postural points for your body, particularly the awareness of grounding with the earth.

As you settle more comfortably into providing this energetic support for your rotating planet, feel an opening at the crown of your head as you also feel an anchoring sensation with the earth below you. In other words, imagine your vertex opening to the heavens allowing vibrations to flow in as you also remain aware of the sensation of the earth and anchoring and holding at your base. As you do whole body (and whole earth and sky) breathing with healing intention you are also allowing the heavens above and the earth under you to support your practice.

At this point become aware of your lower belly. As you inhale see if you can draw energy into this area. As you exhale see if you can have a focus point in this area. Imagine holding your good will intention for the planet in your lower belly and this becomes the center from which energy flows from you through your hands into the earth. Particularly now keep your awareness in the soles of your feet, the palms of your hands, and in your lower belly - all with the intention of the expansive/ contractive force of existence to breathe with and support your planet earth floating between your hands. Do this for several minutes letting whatever happens happen. Then let go of this exercise and relax, embracing your belly with your hands.

There were a lot of words above to describe details of this practice. But once you get it, it is not so complex. It is simply in the beginning, I am giving extra detail (since this is a book, not in person) to insure you have sufficient feel for the practice. Take it slow, don't push yourself too hard, but keep at it over time. Things will settle in and become easier. If they don't become easier, back off, and see what is not working. You may need to adapt sometimes to what feels right for you.

Begin to work with other things than our planet. You could imagine a relative's hurt ankle between your hands, or an aged person who is fatigued, or a hurt kitty, or simply a healthy good friend. In the beginning find those you easily have intention to support and place them in this field between your hands. Bring your star or tree to this space. With time start including those you feel more neutral about, and then those you have more difficulty with intending them well-being. Find the place in you, and in your belly, where your intention and the energetic support through your hands have equanimity, that is that they treat all equally, be it the planet, a friend, a mosquito, or a perceived enemy or evil person. Find the place where you share the same vibrational universe. This is a long term key element to this practice. As you progress keep reminding yourself to KEEP GROUNDED through maintaining awareness of the sensation where your body connects with the chair/floor/ground. *And don't force yourself.*

Recall I've asked you to alternate Exercise #3 with Exercise #2. In #2 you are listening/resonating/harmonizing to find the star in you that shines with the star in the abyss of the heavens. As in same same. You are learning from this connection the star's fundamental activity and intention. In Exercise #3 you are intending that star your natural best with all

your body and breath and spirit. With time
and practice you will find each other, and thus
love itself.

FINAL THOUGHTS ....

This little text is an initial primer to assist you in discovering your Qi dynamic, the activity that unifies you with your world. In essence, the fundamental activity underlying all reality is a constantly reborn cosmic embrace. Once you've got a feel for the experience of this as the fundamental relationship with others, you will be able to deepen connections on your own. Then when you walk, when you sit under a tree, listen to a bird sing, have a drink with a friend, view the night sky; all will be yourself.

As the Diamond Sutra puts it:

A star in the night sky
A bubble on a stream
Lightning in a summer storm
A street lamp on a dark night
A phantom in a dream.

APPENDIX

I provide here an excerpt of the Chinese and the English translation of the "Mu" koan I noted in Chapter 4. It is from the Mumonkan, a text of koans compiled in the 13th century by the Chinese Zen master Wumen Huikai, Japanese Mumon Ekai. This translation is from Kazuki Sekida in his text Two Zen Classics: The Gateless Gate and the Blue Cliff Records.

Case 1 Jōshû's "Mu" 一　趙州狗子

趙州和尚、因僧問、狗子還有佛性也無。州云、無。

A monk asked Jōshû, "Has a dog the Buddha Nature?" Jōshû answered, "Mu."

Mumon's Comment

無門曰、參禪須透祖師關、妙悟要窮心路絶。

In order to master Zen, you must pass the barrier of the patriarchs. To attain this subtle realization, you must completely cut off the way of thinking.

祖關不透心路不絶、盡是依草附木精靈。

If you do not pass the barrier, and do not cut off the way of thinking, then you will be like a ghost clinging to the bushes and weeds.

且道、如何是祖師關。

Now, I want to ask you, what is the barrier of the patriarchs?

只者一箇無字、乃宗門一關也。

Why, it is this single word "Mu." That is the front gate to Zen.

遂目之曰禪宗無門關。

Therefore it is called the "Mumonkan of Zen."

透得過者、非但親見趙州、便可與歷代祖師把手共行、眉毛廝結同一眼見、同一耳聞。

If you pass through it, you will not only see Jōshû face to face, but you will also go hand in hand with the successive patriarchs, entangling your eyebrows with theirs, seeing with the same eyes, hearing with the same ears.

豈不慶快。

Isn't that a delightful prospect?

莫有要透關底麼。

Wouldn't you like to pass this barrier?

將三百六十骨節、八萬四千毫竅、通身起箇疑團參箇無字。

Arouse your entire body with its three hundred and sixty bones and joints and its eighty-four thousand pores of the skin; summon up a spirit of great doubt and concentrate on this word "Mu."

畫夜提撕、莫作虛無會、莫作有無會。

Carry it continuously day and night. Do not form a nihilistic conception of vacancy, or a relative conception of "has" or "has not."

如吞了箇熱鐵丸相似、吐又吐不出。

It will be just as if you swallow a red-hot iron ball, which you cannot spit out even if you try.

蕩盡從　前惡知惡覚、久久純熟自然內外打成一片、如啞子得夢、只許自知。

All the illusory ideas and delusive thoughts accumulated up to the present will be exterminated, and when the time comes, internal and external will be spontaneously united. You will know this, but for yourself only, like a dumb man who has had a dream.

驀然打發、驚天　動地。

Then all of a sudden an explosive conversion will occur, and you will astonish the heavens and shake the earth.

From:

Sekida, Kazuki, (2005). *Two Zen Classics: The Gateless Gate and the Blue Cliff Records*

REFERENCES

Chapter 1
Taylor, Jill Bolte (2008). *Stroke of Insight, a Ted Talk*
https://www.ted.com/talks/
jill_bolte_taylor_my_stroke_of_insight

What the Bleep!? (2006). *Dr. Quantum - Double Slit Experiment*
https://www.youtube.com/watch?v=Q1YqgPAtzho

Chapter 3
Isaacson, Walter (2007). *Einstein: His Life and Universe*, (Chapters 5, 6, 7 & 9). Simon and Schuster.

Chapter 5
Boone, J. Allen (1954). *Kinship with All Life* Harper.

Oschman, James (2000). *Energy Medicine; The Scientific Basis*, (Chapters 2 & 7). Churchhill Livingston.

Biofields, Global Advances in Health (2015).
https://journals.sagepub.com/toc/gama/4/1_suppl

Cohen, Leonard. *Anthem, Come Healing, & Love Itself*.

CONTACT

Thank you for reading. If you have any comments, questions, insights, repercussions, etc, please write. This is the first of likely two or three books on this topic. The next little book will build on the practices and understanding presented here and go more deeply into the physics of the phases of Qi and the emergence of self. So if you'd like updates on future publications and workshops, please contact me to be put on the mailing list.

My email is Physicsofqi@gmail.com.

ABOUT THE AUTHOR

Soko Paul Karsten

Paul is a teacher, curriculum specialist, and practitioner of East Asian Medicine for the last forty years, a Zen monk who started practice and training in 1973, a Qi practitioner for as long as he can remember, and a cosmologist at heart. He resides on a small island in the Philippines where he does research into direct experience of the natural world and its relationship with the dynamic of Qi.

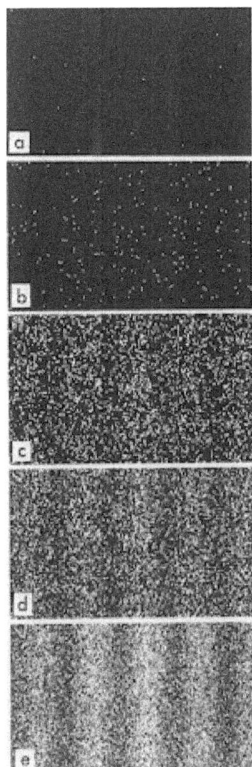

Photons emerge one at a time from their field
to chaotically etch out on a photographic
plate the fundamental activity of the cosmos.
Compliments of the Double Slit Experiment.

www.ingramcontent.com/pod-product-compliance
Lightning Source LLC
Chambersburg PA
CBHW032116280326
41933CB00009B/869